I0701689

FOOD ALLERGIES AND INTOLERANCE

Understanding and managing your condition
through diet

By

DR William A. Robertson

All rights reserved.Copyright ©DR William A . Robertson.

(2023). No part of this publication may be reproduced, distributed, or transmitted in any form or by any means, including photocopying, recording or other electronic, or mechanical methods, without the prior written permission of the publisher, except in the case of brief quotations embodied in critical review and certain other non-commercial uses permitted by copyright law.

TABLE OF CONTENTS

Introduction

Living with a food sensitivity doesn't need to feel overwhelming, unpleasant, or overpowering. When you have a reasonable comprehension of what sets off a response in your body, do whatever it takes to guarantee you stay away from communication no matter what.

The following are a couple of ways of assisting you with dealing with your dinners without living in a feeling of dread toward the fixings.

1.Always read names
 Today, food names incorporate significant sensitivity data, for example, whether any added substances contain milk protein or results of wheat, or whether a food was created in an office that cycles nuts. In any case, you want to peruse each name, without fail — regardless of whether you have bought the thing many times previously. Producers much of the time change fixings and an allergen might be essential for another plan.

2.Take consideration while cooking.
 On the off chance that everybody in the family isn't following a sans allergen diet, you need to make certain

to keep away from cross-defilement. It's really smart to have two arrangements of cooking and eating utensils — one only for the unfavorably susceptible individual — with the goal that a blade used to cut a peanut butter sandwich isn't incidentally squeezed into administration buttering the toast of somebody who's over sensitive to peanuts. All dishes and utensils ought to be completely washed in hot, lathery water between utilizes.

3.Dine out protectively.

It's wise to tell the supervisor or culinary specialist about your food sensitivity before you request. Individuals with food sensitivities frequently convey a culinary expert card — a printed note determining every one of the fixings you are hypersensitive to as well as a solicitation that all dishes, utensils, and planning surfaces be liberated from hints of that food. Drive-through eateries and bistros are no special case. Understand names and pose inquiries prior to choosing what to eat and drink.

4.Formulate an activity plan.

Make a rundown of moves toward take. Would it be a good idea for you to inadvertently eat the food you are oversensitive to, and convey a printed duplicate of the arrangement with you.

5.Wear a clinical ID wristband.

Ensure it records pertinent data about your food sensitivity.

6.Always convey your medicine, in a perfect world two dosages.

Assuming your PCP has recommended crisis medicine for you generally take it with you and consistently convey two to be certain you're ready in the event that you cause problems. Certain individuals with food sensitivities additionally convey allergy meds. Try not to venture out from home without your drugs.

About allergens

Albeit any food can cause an unfavorably susceptible response, there are as of now 14 significant allergens comprising of:

.Milk
.Cereals containing gluten
.Eggs
.Peanuts
.Tree nuts
.Sesame seeds
.Scavengers
.Molluscs
.Fish
.Celery
.Mustard
.Lupin
.Soya
.Sulfur dioxide

Indeed, even small measures of these allergens can cause a response when ingested, contacted or breathed in.

A great deal of food varieties contain these fixings so in the event that you truly do have a response to an allergen, you would need to eliminate the assortment of food you devour, meaning you will not have the option to eat a decent eating routine.

Adjusted abstains from food

Adjusted counts calories comprise of a wide assortment of food varieties eaten in the right extents, and are fundamental for kids' development and improvement, as well as to assist grown-ups with getting every one of the supplements they need for their bodies to appropriately work. There are six classifications of supplements that our bodies need, including protein, starches, fat, nutrients, minerals and water. In any case, when you have food sensitivities, it tends to be hard to track down nutritious and delicious food varieties that don't contain explicit allergens, and giving safe food can be a challenge.

Chapter 1:FOOD SENSITIVITY AND NARROW MINDEDNESS

Individuals frequently have an upsetting response to something they ate and think they have a food sensitivity. In any case, they might be having something different: a response called food narrow mindedness.

What's the distinction?

A food sensitivity is brought about by your insusceptible framework responding to the food as needs be.

With a food prejudice, your safe framework isn't mindful. More often than not it's an issue with processing the food.

For instance, being adversely affected by milk is not quite the same as not having the option to process it appropriately due to lactose bigotry.

Certain individuals come from families where sensitivities are normal - - not really food sensitivities, but rather maybe roughage fever, asthma, or hives. When both of your folks have sensitivities, you're bound to have food sensitivities than if by some stroke of good luck one parent has sensitivities.

How Food Sensitivities Work
Food sensitivities include two pieces of your invulnerable framework. One is immunoglobulin E (IgE), a sort of protein called a neutralizer that travels through the blood. The other is pole cells, which you have in all

body tissues however particularly in places like your nose, throat, lungs, skin, and gastrointestinal system.

Whenever you first eat a food you're sensitive to, certain phones make a great deal of IgE for the piece of the food that sets off your sensitivity, called an allergen. The IgE gets delivered and joins to the outer layer of pole cells. You will not have a response yet, however presently you're set up for one.

The following time you eat that food, the allergen connects with that IgE and triggers the pole cells to deliver synthetic compounds like receptors. Contingent upon the tissue they're in, these synthetics will cause different side effects. What's more, since some food allergens aren't separated by the intensity of cooking or by stomach acids or compounds that digest food, they can cross into your circulatory system. From that point, they can travel and cause unfavorably susceptible responses all through your body.

The absorption interaction influences the timing and the area. You might feel tingling in your mouth. Then you might have side effects like retching, the runs, or midsection torment. Food allergens in your blood can cause a drop in circulatory strain. As they arrive at your skin, they can set off hives or dermatitis. In the lungs, they might cause wheezing. Each of this happens inside a couple of moments to 60 minutes.

Which Food Sensitivities Are Generally Normal?

In grown-ups, they include:

.Peanuts
.Tree nuts, like pecans
.Shellfish, including shrimp, crawfish, . .lobster, and crab

For youngsters, the food allergens that most frequently cause issues are:

Eggs
Milk
Peanuts
Grown-ups generally don't lose their sensitivities, yet kids do in some cases. Kids are bound to grow out of sensitivity to milk, eggs, and soy than to peanuts, fish, and shrimp.
The food sources that you'll respond to are much of the time those that you eat consistently. In Japan, for instance, you'll track down rice sensitivity. In Scandinavia, codfish sensitivity is normal

Side effects
For certain individuals, an unfavorably susceptible response to a specific food might be awkward however not serious. For others, a hypersensitive food response can be terrifying and even dangerous. Food sensitivity side effects as a rule foster inside a couple of moments to 2 hours subsequent to eating the culpable food. Seldom, side effects might be postponed for a few hours.

The most well-known food sensitivity signs and side effects include:
Shivering or tingling in the mouth
Hives, tingling or skin inflammation
Enlarging of the lips, face, tongue and throat or different pieces of the body
Wheezing, nasal blockage or inconvenience relaxing
Stomach torment, looseness of the bowels, sickness or retching
Unsteadiness, discombobulation or swooning

Chapter 2:THE SIGNIFICANT OF A SOUND STOMACH MICROBIOME FOR OVERSEEING FOOD SENSITIVITIES AND PREJUDICE.

Your body is loaded with trillions of microbes, infections and parasites. They are aggregately known as the microbiome.

While certain microorganisms are related with illness, others are quite significant for your safe framework, heart, weight and numerous different parts of wellbeing.

What Is the Stomach Microbiome?

Microscopic organisms, infections, parasites and other infinitesimal living things are alluded to as microorganisms, or microorganisms, for short.
Trillions of these organisms exist primarily inside your digestion tracts and on your skin.
The majority of the organisms in your digestion tracts are viewed as in a "pocket" of your internal organ called the cecum, and they are alluded to as the stomach microbiome.
Albeit various kinds of organisms live inside you, microorganisms are the most examined.

Truth be told, there are more bacterial cells in your body than human cells. There are approximately 40 trillion bacterial cells in your body and just 30 trillion human cells. That implies you are a greater number of microorganisms than human .

Likewise, there depend on 1,000 types of microorganisms in the human stomach microbiome, and every one of them assumes an alternate part in your body. The greater part of them are critical for your wellbeing, while others might cause sickness.

Through and through, these organisms might weigh as much as 2-5 pounds (1-2 kg), which is generally the heaviness of your mind. Together, they capability as an additional organ in your body and assume a tremendous part in your wellbeing.

How Can It Influence Your Body?

People have developed to live with organisms for a long period of time.
During this time, organisms have figured out how to assume vital parts in the human body. As a matter of fact, without the stomach microbiome, it would be undeniably challenging to get by.

The stomach microbiome starts to influence your body the second you are conceived.

You are first presented to microorganisms when you go through your mom's introduction to the world channel. Nonetheless, new proof proposes that children might interact for certain organisms while inside the belly.

As you develop, your stomach microbiome starts to broaden, meaning it begins to contain various kinds of microbial species. Higher microbiome variety is viewed as really great for your wellbeing.
Curiously, the food you eat influences the variety of your stomach microbes.

As your microbiome develops, it influences your body in various ways, including:
Processing bosom milk: A portion of the microbes that initially start to develop inside children's digestive organs are called Bifidobacteria. They digest the sound sugars in bosom milk that are significant for development (8, 9, 10).
Processing fiber: Certain microscopic organisms digest fiber, delivering short-chain unsaturated fats, which are

significant for stomach wellbeing. Fiber might assist with forestalling weight gain, diabetes, coronary illness and the gamble of malignant growth.

Helping control your invulnerable framework: The stomach microbiome likewise controls how your insusceptible framework functions. By speaking with insusceptible cells, the stomach microbiome have some control over how your body answers disease.

Assisting control with braining wellbeing: New exploration recommends that the stomach microbiome may likewise influence the focal sensory system, which controls mind capability.

Subsequently, there are various manners by which the stomach microbiome can influence key physical processes and impact your wellbeing.

1.

There are great many various kinds of microbes in your digestive organs, the majority of which benefit your wellbeing.
Notwithstanding, having an excessive number of undesirable organisms can prompt sickness.
A lopsidedness of sound and undesirable organisms is once in a while called stomach dysbiosis, and it might add to weight gain.

A few notable examinations have shown that the stomach microbiome varied totally between indistinguishable twins, one of whom had heftiness and one of whom didn't. This showed that distinctions in the microbiome were not hereditary.

Curiously, in one review, when the microbiome from the twin with heftiness was moved to mice, they put on more weight those that had gotten the microbiome of the other twin, notwithstanding the two gatherings eating a similar eating regimen .

These examinations show that microbiome dysbiosis may assume a part in weight gain.
Luckily, probiotics are great for a solid microbiome and can assist with weight reduction. By the by, studies propose that the impacts of probiotics on weight reduction are presumably tiny, with individuals losing under 2.2 pounds

2. It Influences Stomach Wellbeing
The microbiome can likewise influence stomach wellbeing and may assume a part in gastrointestinal illnesses like crabby entrail condition (IBS) and fiery gut sickness (IBD) .

The swelling, spasms and stomach torment that individuals with IBS experience might be because of stomach dysbiosis. This is on the grounds that the microorganisms produce a ton of gas and different synthetic substances, which add to the side effects of digestive uneasiness.

Be that as it may, certain solid microscopic organisms in the microbiome can likewise further develop stomach wellbeing.
Certain Bifidobacteria and Lactobacilli, which are tracked down in probiotics and yogurt, can assist with fixing holes between gastrointestinal cells and forestall defective stomach condition.

These species can likewise forestall infection causing microscopic organisms from adhering to the gastrointestinal wall.
Truth be told, taking specific probiotics that contain Bifidobacteria and Lactobacilli can diminish side effects of IBS .

3.The Stomach Microbiome Might Help Heart Wellbeing
Curiously, the stomach microbiome may try and influence heart wellbeing.
A new report in 1,500 individuals found that the stomach microbiome assumed a significant part in advancing "great" HDL cholesterol and fatty substances
Certain unfortunate species in the stomach microbiome may likewise add to coronary illness by creating trimethylamine N-oxide (TMAO).

TMAO is a synthetic that adds to obstructed corridors, which might prompt respiratory failures or stroke.

Certain microorganisms inside the microbiome convert choline and L-carnitine, the two of which are supplements found in red meat and other creature based food sources, to TMAO, possibly expanding risk factors for coronary illness .

Nonetheless, different microorganisms inside the stomach microbiome, especially Lactobacilli, may assist with decreasing cholesterol when taken as a probiotic.

HOW CAN YOU FURTHER DEVELOP YOUR STOMACH MICROBIOME?

There are numerous ways of further developing your stomach microbiome, including:

1.Eat a different scope of food sources: This can prompt an assorted microbiome, which is a sign of good stomach wellbeing. Specifically, vegetables, beans and organic product contain bunches of fiber and can advance the development of sound Bifidobacteria .

2.Eat aged food varieties:
Matured food varieties like yogurt, sauerkraut and kefir all contain sound microorganisms, predominantly Lactobacilli, and can lessen how much sickness causing species in the stomach.

3.Limit your admission of fake sugars: Some proof has shown that counterfeit sugars like aspartame increment glucose by animating the development of undesirable microorganisms like Enterobacteriaceae in the stomach microbiome.

4.Eat prebiotic food sources:
Prebiotics are a kind of fiber that invigorates the development of sound microorganisms. Prebiotic-rich food varieties incorporate artichokes, bananas, asparagus, oats and apples.

5.Breastfeed for somewhere around a half year:
Breastfeeding is vital for the improvement of the stomach microbiome. Youngsters who are breastfed for somewhere around a half year have more useful Bifidobacteria than the individuals who are bottle-taken care of.

6.Eat entire grains:
Entire grains contain loads of fiber and valuable carbs like beta-glucan, which are processed by stomach microscopic organisms to help weight, malignant growth chance, diabetes and different issues.

7.Attempt a plant-based diet:
Veggie lover diets might assist with decreasing degrees of infection causing microscopic organisms like E. coli, as well as irritation and cholesterol.

8.Eat food sources rich in polyphenols: Polyphenols are plant intensifies tracked down in red wine, green tea, dull chocolate, olive oil and entire grains. They are separated by the microbiome to invigorate solid bacterial development.

9.Take a probiotic supplement:
Probiotics are live microbes that can assist with reestablishing the stomach to a sound state after dysbiosis. They do this by "reseeding" it with solid microorganisms.

10.Take anti-toxins just when important:
Anti-microbials kill numerous terrible and great microscopic organisms in the stomach microbiome, conceivably adding to weight gain and anti-infection obstruction. Along these lines, possibly take anti-infection agents when medicinally essential.

CHAPTER 3: HOW TO TRANSIT TO A SAFE SOLID EATING ROUTINE:

1.Slow down
 The speed at which you eat impacts the amount you eat, as well as the fact that you are so prone to put on weight.

As a matter of fact, concentrates on looking at changed eating speeds show that quick eaters are considerably more liable to eat more and have a higher weight file (BMI) than slow eaters.

Your hunger, the amount you eat, and how full you get are completely constrained by chemicals. Chemicals sign to your cerebrum whether you're eager or full.

In any case, it requires around 20 minutes for your cerebrum to get these messages. That is the reason eating all the more leisurely may give your cerebrum the time it necessities to see that you're full.

Studies have affirmed this, showing that eating gradually may diminish the quantity of calories you consume at feasts and assist you with getting thinner.

Eating gradually is likewise connected to more careful biting, which has additionally been connected to further developed weight control.

Thus, essentially eating increasingly slow more frequently may assist you with eating less.

2. **Pick entire grain bread rather than refined.**
You can without much of a stretch make your eating routine a piece better by picking entire grain bread instead of conventional refined grain bread.

Refined grains have been related with numerous medical problems. Entire grains, then again, have been connected to an assortment of medical advantages, including a decreased gamble of type 2 diabetes, coronary illness, and malignant growth

They're likewise a decent wellspring of:

fiber
B nutrients
minerals like zinc, iron, magnesium, and manganese.

There are numerous assortments of entire grain bread accessible, and a significant number of them even taste better compared to refined bread.

Simply make a point to peruse the mark to guarantee that your bread is made with entire grains just, not a combination of entire and refined grains. It's additionally ideal that the bread contains entire seeds or grains.

3. **Add Greek yogurt to your eating routine**
Greek yogurt (or Greek-style yogurt) is thicker and creamier than normal yogurt.

It has been stressed to eliminate its overabundance whey, which is the watery piece of milk. This outcomes in an end result that is higher in fat and protein than ordinary yogurt.

As a matter of fact, it contains up to two times as much protein as a similar measure of customary yogurt does, or as much as 10 grams for every 3.5 ounces.

Eating a decent wellspring of protein can assist you with feeling more full for longer, which can assist with dealing with your hunger and decrease your food consumption, assuming that is your objective.

Besides, since Greek yogurt has been stressed, it contains less carbs and less lactose than standard yogurt. This makes it reasonable for individuals who follow a low carb diet or are lactose prejudiced.

Essentially supplant a few bites or normal yogurt assortments with Greek yogurt for a generous portion of protein and supplements.

Simply make a point to pick the plain, unflavored assortments. Seasoned yogurts might be loaded with added sugar and other less nutritious fixings.

4. **Try not to shop without a rundown**
There are two significant systems to utilize when you go shopping for food: Make your shopping list early and don't go to the store hungry.

Not knowing precisely very thing you really want accounts for drive purchasing, while yearning can make you throw considerably more low supplement food sources into your shopping basket.

That is the reason the best technique is to prepare and record what you want ahead of time. By doing this and adhering to your rundown, you'll not just purchase better things to keep around the house, yet you'll likewise set aside cash.

5. Eat eggs, ideally for breakfast
Eggs are unimaginably sound, particularly assuming you eat them toward the beginning of the day.

They are wealthy in great protein and numerous fundamental supplements that individuals frequently don't get enough of, like choline.

While seeing investigations looking at different kinds of calorie-matched morning meals, eggs prove to be the best.

Eating eggs in the first part of the day builds sensations of completion. This has been displayed to make individuals consume less calories at later dinners. It tends to be very useful for weight reduction, assuming that is your objective.

For instance, one concentrate in 50 individuals found that having an egg-based breakfast diminished sensations of craving and diminished how much calories consumed later in the day than a morning meal of grain.

Thus, essentially supplanting your ongoing breakfast with eggs might bring about significant advantages for your wellbeing.

6. **Increment your protein admission**

Protein is frequently alluded to as the lord of supplements, and it appears to have a few superpowers.

Because of its capacity to influence your appetite and satiety chemicals, it's not unexpected considered the most filling of the macronutrients.

One review showed that eating a high-protein feast diminished degrees of ghrelin, the craving chemical, in excess of a high-carb dinner in individuals with weight.

Additionally, protein assists you with holding bulk and may likewise marginally build the quantity of calories you consume each day. It's additionally significant for forestalling the deficiency of bulk that can happen with weight reduction and as you age.

On the off chance that you're attempting to get more fit, expect to add a wellspring of protein to every dinner and tidbit. It will assist you with feeling more full for longer, control desires, and make you less inclined to indulge.

Great wellsprings of protein include:

dairy items

nuts
peanut butter
eggs
beans
lean meat

7. **Hydrate**

Drinking sufficient water is significant for your wellbeing.

Many examinations have demonstrated the way that drinking water can increment weight reduction and advance weight upkeep, and it might try and somewhat increment the quantity of calories you consume every day.

Concentrates additionally demonstrate the way that drinking water before feasts can lessen your craving and food admission during the accompanying dinner.

All things considered, the main thing is to hydrate rather than different drinks. This may radically diminish your admission of sugar and calories.

Drinking water consistently may likewise be connected to further developed diet quality and could diminish your calorie consumption from refreshments.

8. **Prepare or broil as opposed to barbecuing or searing**

The manner in which you set up your food can radically change its consequences for your wellbeing.

Barbecuing, cooking, broiling, and profound searing are famous techniques for getting ready meat and fish.

In any case, during these sorts of cooking strategies, a few possibly harmful mixtures are framed. These incorporate:

polycyclic fragrant hydrocarbons
high level glycation finished results
heterocyclic amines
These mixtures have been connected to a few medical issue, including malignant growth and coronary illness (34Trusted Source, 35Trusted Source, 36Trusted Source).

Better cooking strategies include:

baking
searing
poaching
pressure cooking
stewing
slow cooking
stewing
sous-vide
These strategies don't advance the arrangement of these destructive mixtures and may make your food better.

In spite of the fact that you can in any case partake in a periodic barbecued or broiled dish, it's ideal to sparingly utilize those techniques.

9. **Take omega-3 and vitamin D** enhancements
Roughly 1 billion individuals all over the planet are lacking in vitamin D.

Vitamin D is a fat-solvent nutrient that is vital for bone wellbeing and the legitimate working of your resistant framework. As a matter of fact, each cell in your body has a receptor for vitamin D, showing its significance.

Vitamin D is tracked down in not very many food varieties, however greasy fish for the most part contains the most noteworthy sums.

Omega-3 unsaturated fats are one more generally deficient with regards to supplement that is tracked down in greasy fish. These play numerous significant parts in the body, including decreasing irritation, keeping up with heart wellbeing, and advancing appropriate mind capability.

The Western eating routine is for the most part exceptionally high in omega-6 unsaturated fats, which increment aggravation and have been connected to numerous ongoing illnesses. Omega-3s assist with battling this irritation and keep your body in a more adjusted state.

In the event that you don't eat greasy fish consistently, you ought to think about taking an enhancement. Omega-3s and vitamin D can frequently be tracked down together in many enhancements.

10. Supplant your number one drive-through joint

Eating out doesn't need to include undesirable food varieties.

Consider overhauling your number one drive-through joint to one with better choices.

There are numerous sound drive-through eateries and combination kitchens offering solid and heavenly dinners.

They may simply be an incredible substitution for your number one burger or pizza place. Likewise, you can by and large get these dinners at an exceptionally respectable cost.

11. Attempt no less than one new solid recipe each week

Choosing what to have for supper can be a consistent reason for dissatisfaction, which is the reason many individuals will generally utilize similar recipes over and over. Odds are good that you've been cooking similar recipes on autopilot for quite a long time.

Whether these are sound or unfortunate recipes, having a go at something new can be a pleasant method for adding greater variety to your eating regimen.

Intend to have a go at making another solid recipe something like one time each week. This can switch around your food and supplement admissions and ideally add a few new and nutritious recipes to your daily practice.

On the other hand, attempt to make a better rendition of a most loved recipe by exploring different avenues regarding new fixings, spices, and flavors.

12. **Pick prepared potatoes over french fries**
Potatoes are very filling and a typical side to many dishes. All things considered, the strategy in which they're arranged to a great extent decides their effect on wellbeing.

First of all, 3.5 ounces (100 grams) of heated potatoes contain 93 calories, while similar measure of french fries contains north of 3 times as many (333 calories) Moreover, southern style french fries for the most part contain destructive mixtures like aldehydes

Supplanting your french fries with heated or bubbled potatoes is an incredible method for shaving off calories and keep away from these undesirable mixtures.

13. **Eat your greens first**

An effective method for guaranteeing that you eat your greens is to appreciate them as a starter.

Thusly, you'll undoubtedly complete your greens while you're all at your hungriest. This might make you eat less of other, maybe less solid, parts of the dinner later. It might lead you to eat less and better calories by and large, which could bring about weight reduction.

Besides, eating vegetables before a carb-rich dinner has been displayed to usefully affect glucose levels.
It dials back the speed at which carbs are retained into the circulation system and may help both short-and long haul glucose control in individuals with diabetes.

14. **Eat your organic products as opposed to drinking them**

Organic products are stacked with water, fiber, nutrients, and cell reinforcements.
Studies have over and over connected eating organic product to a decreased gamble of a few medical issue, like coronary illness, type 2 diabetes, and disease.

Since organic products contain fiber and different plant compounds, their regular sugars are by and large processed gradually and don't cause significant spikes in glucose levels.

In any case, the equivalent doesn't have any significant bearing to organic product juices.

Many organic product juices aren't even produced using genuine natural product, but instead concentrate and sugar. A few assortments might try and contain as much sugar as a sweet soda

Indeed, even genuine natural product juices miss the mark on fiber and biting obstruction given by entire organic products. This makes organic product squeeze considerably more prone to spike your glucose levels, driving you to consume a lot in a solitary sitting.

15. Cook at home on a more regular basis

Attempt to make a propensity for cooking at home most evenings as opposed to eating out.
As far as one might be concerned, it's more straightforward on your spending plan.

Second, by preparing your food yourself, you'll know precisely exact thing is in it. You will not need to ponder any secret unfortunate or unhealthy fixings.
Likewise, by cooking huge servings, you'll likewise have extras for the following day, guaranteeing a good feast then, at that point, as well.

At long last, cooking at home has been related with a lower hazard of weight and further developed diet quality, particularly among youngsters

16. Turn out to be more dynamic

Great sustenance and exercise frequently remain inseparable. Practice has been displayed to work on your mind-set, as well as abatement sensations of misery, uneasiness, and stress.

These are the specific sentiments that are probably going to add to close to home and voraciously consuming food
Beside reinforcing your muscles and bones, exercise might help you
get more fit
increment your energy levels
decrease your gamble of ongoing infections
work on your rest

Expect to do around 30 minutes of moderate to extreme focus practice every day, or just use the stairwell and continue short strolls whenever the situation allows.

17. **Supplant sweet drinks with shimmering water**
Sweet refreshments could be the unhealthiest thing you can drink.
They're stacked with added sugar, which has been connected to various sicknesses, including
coronary illness
stoutness
type 2 diabetes

Also, the additional sugar found in these beverages doesn't affect hunger the same way as normal food does. This implies you don't make up for the calories you drink by eating any less

One 16-ounce (492-ml) sweet soft drink contains around 207 calories

Have a go at supplanting your sweet drink with either a sans sugar elective or basically pick still or shining water all things being equal. Doing so will shave off the non-advantageous calories and lessen your admission of abundance sugar.

18. **Avoid "diet" food sources**

Purported diet food sources can very mislead. They have typically had their fat substance decreased emphatically and are frequently marked "without fat," "low fat," "fat-diminished," or "low calorie."

In any case, to make up for the lost flavor and surface from fat, sugar and different fixings are frequently added.

In this way, many eating routine food sources wind up containing more sugar and here and there much a larger number of calories than their full fat partners

All things being equal, choose entire food varieties like products of the soil.

19. **Get a decent night's rest**

The significance of good rest couldn't possibly be more significant.

Lack of sleep upsets hunger guidelines, frequently prompting expanded craving. This outcomes in expanded calorie admission and weight gain

As a matter of fact, individuals who rest excessively minimal will generally weigh essentially more than the people who get sufficient rest

Being restless additionally adversely influences fixation, efficiency, athletic execution, glucose digestion, and resistant capability.

Additionally, it builds your gamble of a few infections, including provocative circumstances and coronary illness
That is the reason it means a lot to attempt to get sufficient measures of good-quality rest, ideally in one session.

20. **Eat new berries rather than dried ones**
Berries are exceptionally sound and loaded with supplements, fiber, and cancer prevention agents. Most assortments can be bought new, frozen, or dried. Albeit numerous types are moderately solid, the dried assortments are a significantly more focused wellspring of calories and sugar, since all the water has been eliminated.

A **3.5-ounce** (**100-gram**) serving of new or frozen strawberries contains 31-35 calories, while 3.5 ounces (100 grams) of dried strawberries contain an incredible 375 calories
The dried assortments are additionally frequently covered with sugar, further expanding the sugar content.

By picking the new assortments, you will get a lot juicier tidbit that is lower in sugar and contains less calories.

21. Choose popcorn instead of chips

It may be surprising that popcorn is a whole grain that's loaded with nutrients and fiber.

A 3.5-ounce (100-gram) serving of air-popped popcorn contains 387 calories and 15 grams of fiber, while the same amount of potato chips contains 532 calories and only 3 grams of fiber

Diets rich in whole grains have been linked to health benefits, such as a reduced risk of inflammation and heart disease.

For a healthy snack, try making your own popcorn at home (not microwave popcorn varieties) or purchase air-popped popcorn.

Many commercial varieties prepare their popcorn with fat, sugar, and salt, making it no healthier than potato chips.

22. Choose healthy oils

Highly processed seed and vegetable oils have become a household staple over the past few decades.

Examples include soybean, cottonseed, sunflower, and canola oils.

These oils are high in omega-6 fatty acids but low in heart-healthy omega-3s.

Some research suggests a high omega-6 to omega-3 ratio can lead to inflammation and has been linked to chronic conditions, such as heart disease, cancer, osteoporosis, and autoimmune disorders

Swap these oils for healthier alternatives, such as:
extra virgin olive oil
avocado oil
coconut oil

23. **Eat from smaller plates**

It has been proven that the size of your dinnerware can affect how much you eat.
Eating from a large plate can make your portion look smaller, while eating from a small plate can make it look bigger.

According to one study, eating from a smaller plate was associated with increased feelings of satiety and reduced energy intake among participants with a healthy body weight

Also, if you don't realize that you're eating more than usual, you won't compensate by eating less at the next meal
By eating from smaller dinnerware, you can trick your brain into thinking that you're eating more, making yourself less likely to overeat.

24. **Get the salad dressing on the side**

Simply getting to the point of being able to order a salad at a restaurant is a great achievement for many.

However, not all salads are equally healthy. In fact, some salads are smothered in high calorie dressings, which may make the salads even higher in calories than other items on the menu.

Asking for the dressing on the side makes it a lot easier to control the portion size and amount of calories that you consume.

25. **Drink your coffee black**

Coffee, which is one of the most popular beverages in the world, is very healthy.
In fact, it's a major source of antioxidants and has been linked to many health benefits, such as a lower risk of type 2 diabetes, mental decline, and liver disease.

However, many commercial varieties of coffee contain lots of additional ingredients, such as sugar, syrup, heavy cream, and sweeteners.
Drinking these varieties quickly negates all of coffee's health benefits and instead adds lots of extra sugar and calories.
Instead, try drinking your coffee black or just adding a small amount of milk or cream instead of sugar.

CHAPTER 4. GLUTEN FREE, DIARY FREE AND SOY FREE RECIPES

QUINOA SALAD

Ingredients:
1 cup quinoa, rinsed
2 cups water
1 cup cherry tomatoes, halved
1 cucumber, diced
1/2 red onion, finely chopped
1/4 cup fresh parsley, chopped
1/4 cup olive oil
2 tablespoons lemon juice
Salt and pepper to taste

Instructions:
In a medium saucepan, combine quinoa and water.
Bring to a boil, then reduce heat to low, cover, and
simmer for 15 minutes, or until quinoa is cooked and
water is absorbed.
Fluff the quinoa with a fork and let it cool to room
temperature.

In a large bowl, combine the cooked quinoa, cherry tomatoes, cucumber, red onion, and parsley.
In a small bowl, whisk together olive oil, lemon juice, salt, and pepper.
Pour the dressing over the quinoa mixture and toss to combine.
Refrigerate for at least 30 minutes before serving to allow the flavors to meld.
Enjoy your gluten-free, soy-free, and dairy-free quinoa salad:

STRAWBERRY SMOOTHIES

How to Make Strawberries Smoothies
These strawberry smoothies are easy to make. They're surprisingly filling, since they offer a good amount of protein and fiber. Whip them up for breakfast, or any time you're in the mood for ice cream—they're that good.

Frozen strawberries offer characteristic berry flavor, antioxidants and a fun pink color. One 10-ounce bag or about 2 cups will be just right. If possible, buy organic strawberries as conventional berries are notoriously high in pesticide exposure.

Frozen bananas make this smoothie lusciously creamy and naturally sweet.

Almond butter offers extra creaminess, plus protein, fiber and heart-healthy monounsaturated fat.

Vanilla almond milk makes this smoothie as creamy as possible (cashew or coconut milk options work well, too). Buy unsweetened to avoid refined sugar. My favorite brands are Malk, Three Trees and Forager's. Or use water, for a slightly less luxurious texture.

For a sweeter smoothie, add maple syrup, to taste. The bananas are typically sweet enough for me, but a little drizzle of maple syrup makes this smoothie taste like a milkshake.

For extra sticking power, you can add up to 1/4 cup old-fashioned oats and/or up to 2 tablespoons flax seed (whole or ground). Flax makes leftover smoothies almost pudding-like in texture.

CHAPTER 5 SUPPORTIVE LIFESTYLE PRACTICES

You can't change your genes, or even much of the environment around you, but there are lifestyle choices you can make to boost your health. Being informed and intentional about diet, activity, sleep, or smoking can reduce your health risks and potentially add years to your life.

1.GETTING THE RIGHT AMOUNT OF SLEEP

Getting the right amount of sleep, and doing so regularly, is first on the list. It's often missed because people focus on diet and exercise, but the link between sleep and life expectancy is supported by research. What surprises some people is that the relationship is a U-shaped curve. This means that too little and too much sleep can affect your lifespan.

A good night's sleep is important to recharge both the body and mind. It helps the body repair cells and get rid of wastes. It also is important in making memories, and sleep deprivation leads to forgetfulness.

Even if you intend to sleep well, health issues can disrupt your plan. Sleep apnea, for example, can greatly increase health risks.

Sleep apnea affects millions of people, but it's believed that many cases are being missed. Part of the reason is that symptoms like snoring, or waking up gasping for air, don't happen in every case. Sleep apnea can present with a number of surprising signs and symptoms, such as teeth grinding and depression.

If you have any concerns, talk to your healthcare provider about a sleep study. There are treatments, like CPAP, that lower risk and improve quality of life. Changes in your sleep patterns can signal other health issues too, so see your healthcare provider for a checkup if anything changes.

2. **EATING Great Equilibrium Dinner**

A sound eating regimen gives you energy and brings down your gamble for coronary illness, diabetes, malignant growth, and different infections. A portion of these circumstances have demonstrated connections to food and nourishment, just like with red meat and colorectal cancer.3

Moving toward a long lasting change in diet will assist more than hopping on the most recent prevailing fashion with eating less junk food does. You might have heard creator Michael Pollan's unmistakable expression: "Eat food. Not to an extreme. Generally plants." Of those plants, pick a rainbow of varieties to ensure you get every one of the supplements you want.

One spot to start is with the very much respected Mediterranean eating routine. It's wealthy in a large number of the best food sources and normally restricts less solid decisions. The more you follow the Mediterranean eating routine, the lower your gamble of a large group of sicknesses

The Mediterranean eating routine has a great deal of leafy foods, entire grains, "great" oils, and a lot of spices and flavors. It doesn't have profoundly handled food varieties, refined grains, or added sugar

3.MAKING TIME FOR ACTIVE WORK

Thirty minutes per day of active work safeguards heart wellbeing. It additionally brings down how much bone misfortune as you age, and with it the gamble of osteoporosis. It's vital to the point that a 2021 investigation of colon malignant growth survivors viewed that as living in a "green" local area that is cordial for practice diminished the gamble of death.5
The best part is that actual work is a minimal expense method for supporting your wellbeing and even set aside you cash. In some cases your wellbeing might restrict your activity choices, yet you can continue moving by washing your windows, cutting your grass, clearing a walkway, and other essential undertakings.

When you are previous age 65, you might benefit by adding equilibrium and adaptability works out, yet continue to move as well. Whether you dance, nursery, swim, or go trekking, pick moderate-force practice that you realize you'll appreciate.

4.KEEPING A SOUND BODY WEIGHT

Stoutness is related with a more limited life expectancy and a higher gamble of numerous illnesses. Fortunately being to some degree overweight doesn't decrease your life span. As a matter of fact, for those over age 65, being on the high side of ordinary than the low side is better.

A recent report saw weight record (BMI) and mortality over a time of 24 years.7 A BMI considered somewhere in the range of 19 and 24 is thought of "typical" or solid. For the people who were in the reach delegated stoutness, a BMI of 30 to 35 implied a 27% increment in mortality. A BMI of 35 to 40 was connected to a 93% expansion.

Among those with a BMI in the overweight territory (BMI 25 to 30), mortality was just higher among the people who smoked. Individuals with a BMI on the high side of ordinary (BMI 24, for instance) had the most minimal demise gambles.

There isn't any genuine sorcery with regards to keeping a solid weight. Eating a nutritious eating regimen and it are the valid "secret" for the vast majority to everyday work-out. Assuming you're battling, talk with your medical services supplier. In any case, remember that prevailing fashion eats less carbs don't work, and your most prominent expectation for progress lies in rolling out long haul improvements.

5. NOT SMOKING OR BITING TOBACCO

Smoking records for nearly 480,000 passings each year in the US alone.8 Added to this are another 16 million individuals who are alive yet adapting to a smoking-related illness.9 In the event that you believe the opportunity should live well for whatever length of time you live, don't smoke or bite tobacco.

The rundown of infections and diseases connected to smoking is long. In the event that you're finding it hard to stop, and you think disease comes just further down the road, it might assist with considering all the more transient objectives. Maybe it's excessively costly, or indoor smoking boycotts limit your social excursions.

Or on the other hand perhaps the midlife concerns will help you! Smoking velocities up wrinkling of the skin. There's likewise a connection among smoking and erectile brokenness in men. Stopping, or keeping away from tobacco in any case, will save lives however safeguard its quality as well.

6. RESTRICTING OR KEEPING AWAY FROM LIQUOR

In spite of the promotion over red wine and life span, liquor ought to be utilized exclusively with some restraint, and for some individuals, not the least bit. Red wine has been found to offer some defensive wellbeing impacts, however there are alternate ways of getting these advantages.

Red wine is wealthy in flavonoids, especially the supplement resveratrol. Resveratrol, be that as it may, is additionally tracked down in red grapes themselves, in red grape squeeze, and even peanuts.

Moderate liquor utilization (one beverage each day for ladies, two for men) may bring down coronary illness risk. However a connection among liquor and bosom disease recommends that even this sum ought to be utilized with alert.

Ladies who have three beverages each week have a 15% higher gamble of bosom disease and the gamble increases another 10% for each extra beverage they have each day.10

More elevated levels of liquor can prompt wellbeing and different issues, including a more serious gamble for:

Stroke
Hypertension
Coronary illness
A few tumors
Mishaps
Savagery
Self destruction
Moderate admission of liquor might be essential for a solid way of life in exceptional minutes, as long as you have no private or family issues with liquor misuse. However long everybody comprehends the dangers, there are times you might drink a toast to your great wellbeing.

Thanks for reading. and more importantly thanks for getting this book.

www.ingramcontent.com/pod-product-compliance
Lightning Source LLC
Chambersburg PA
CBHW071008260726

48661CB00007B/2855